20 EXERCISES FC

20 EXERCISES FOR GREAT LEGS

Your complete shape-up plan

Julia Swift

THORSONS PUBLISHING GROUP

First published in 1989

British Library Cataloguing in Publication Data

Swift, Julia
    20 exercises for great legs.
    1. Man. legs. Muscles. Exercises
    I. Title
    613.7'11

    ISBN 0-7225-1799-8

Photographs © Martin Brigdale

Published by Thorsons Publishers Limited,
Wellingborough, Northamptonshire NN8 2RQ, England

Typeset by Burns & Smith, Derby
Printed in Great Britain by Woolnough Bookbinding Limited,
Irthlingborough, Northamptonshire

10   9   8   7   6   5   4   3   2   1

CONTENTS

ACKNOWLEDGEMENTS

I couldn't have put this book together without the help of a lot of people. I would like to thank them all and to thank Reebok for providing the shoes, Crait for Sam's leotards, Spenco for the weights and Burlingtons for taming Sam's hair.

Special thanks must go to Samantha Shinner for being a 'model' model, to my photographer Martin Brigdale and to Thorsons for turning it all into reality.

Finally I must thank all my students, either at the Brighton or London Studios, who have inspired me and kept me on my toes.

INTRODUCTION

Are you ashamed of your legs? Do you ever yearn for firm, shapely and unforgettable legs? Have you done every exercise under the sun and still not seen results? If you have answered just one 'yes' then *20 Exercises for Great Legs* is for you.

Failure in the past may have stemmed from an imbalance in your exercise programme and poor exercise technique. Read this book, put theory into practise and you will achieve your goal — legs firm and well defined, shapely calves and trim ankles. The results you want will only come by doing your homework now — read the instructions and study the photographs carefully and make exercise a regular slot in your lifestyle.

Spot reducing

It's important to remember that spot reducing — burning fat from specific areas — is not possible. Nor can you add inches to the length of your legs or change your basic structure. It is also a sad fact that thighs and hips for women tend to be sites for accumulated fat. However, the good news is that you can lose excess pounds (and it will be from all over the body) if you follow a well-balanced diet and expend more energy with aerobic-type activities.

Pick your own balance by mixing and matching

You can control and zero in on your body's weak spots and design a body to be proud of. Balancing your exercise quota with different forms of exercise means you're more assured of success than if you concentrate on only one type.

Your mixing and matching streamlining plan should regularly feature (at least three times a week) aerobic activity such as brisk walking, running, swimming and cycling. When partnered with these specially designed exercises, which work on specific muscle groups, a lot can be done to improve and recontour your legs, so that they become shapelier and firmer.

By allowing yourself an hour, at the most, for warming up, exercise and warming down you should be able to create for yourself a programme that only takes a few hours a week.

Apart from a balanced mixture, your programme should be balanced in content. Strengthening or toning-type exercises should be partnered with stretching exercises to gain maximum effect. You will find these specially designed stretch exercises on pages 35–39 and 55–62. Also, the amount of exercise you give one specific muscle group should be equal to that given to its opposing group. For example, when you work on the front of your thighs, pay equal attention to the back of your thighs, too.

TAKING A CLOSER LOOK AT WHICH MUSCLES YOU WILL BE EXERCISING

The quadriceps
(the muscles at the front of your thighs)

Each quadricep is a four-part muscle lying between hip and knee and is the principle shaper of your thigh. It also supplies much of the power needed to run, kick, lift or push. Strong, healthy quadricep muscles are important in protecting your vulnerable knee joints. They also make it easier to help lift heavy objects, rather than lifting incorrectly and using your back muscles.

An effective way to strengthen these muscles is to bend and straighten your leg at the knee joint. If, however, you have an existing knee injury, another way is to lift the leg straight up and down. See exercises on pages 30, 41, 42.

The hamstrings
(the muscles at the back of your thighs)

Opposing the front is a three-part muscle that works together with a major buttock muscle — the gluteus maximus. For your exercising efforts to be truly effective it is important that you balance out the amount of exercising the opposing muscle groups at the front and back of the thighs get. It is all too easy to concentrate on the front because it is always in your line of vision!

You can exercise the hamstrings by either bending your leg at the knee and bringing your foot back up to your bottom, or you can involve your buttock muscles more by taking your leg out behind you, and, in some of the exercises you will feel your buttock muscles working, too.

While many experts agree that strong abdominal muscles help to maintain good posture and help prevent some back pain, they also agree that strong hamstring and buttock muscles also reduce the risk of back problems — and you have the added bonus of a wonderful looking bottom! See exercises on pages 43 and 44.

The abductors (the muscles at the outside of your thighs and hips)

These muscles work as a team. They lift your leg away from your body and also rotate it. They help in everyday movements such as walking and standing as they stabilize the hip joint.

When you exercise this area, correct positioning is vital for full effectiveness. Always make sure your hips, knees and ankles are facing square to the front, otherwise you will work the front of your thighs. Start by lying down and do the classic straight leg lift. Later, add the bent lift version. See exercises on pages 46 and 48.

The adductors (your inside thigh muscles)

Apart from looking more defined and shapelier, well-conditioned inner thighs will help you improve other activities such as running, as they ensure that your legs move in a straight line and increase stability.

To make the exercises more effective, use a ball or cushion to squeeze against as you lie on your back. This position is sometimes the best solution for people with back problems.

When you are ready to progress, and as long as you have the flexibility to get into and maintain the position, use the inner thigh lift. See exercises on pages 49 and 50.

Your lower legs

In the quest for great legs, 100 per cent attention is usually given to thighs and their partners hips and buttocks, but spare a thought for your hardworking lower legs. Now that your attention is caught, you probably zeroed-in on your calves. But what about your shins? Perhaps because they play no major part in the shape of your legs they are often overlooked. However, to minimize the risk of muscle imbalance and injury it is important to increase their strength. There is also the bonus of stronger ankles. See exercise on page 51.

Calves
(gastrocnemius and soleus muscles)

Not only do attractive and shapely calves make your legs even more unforgettable, but the muscles have a functional use as well. They are needed for activities like running, walking and jumping. However, it is a sad fact that wearing high heels to show off and enhance a shapely leg can contribute to an eventual *loss* of shape as they limit calf action. The best remedy is to save high heels for special occasions and practise the heel raise exercise and stretching frequently. See exercises on pages 52 and 53.

TECHNIQUE TIPS

When done correctly the exercises in this book are marvellous for re-contouring your legs but can become worthless and occasionally even harmful when practised incorrectly.

With any exercise, correct positioning and alignment are the key to success. Since most of the thigh muscles extend to the hips and pelvis it's not surprising then that the lower back and hips can fall foul of poor technique and overwork — especially when first starting out.

For each exercise I have included tips and hints to help overcome these problems. A 'popular' mistake is with body alignment and incorrect starting positions. Another is trying to do too much, too soon and too fast! The following hints should go a long way to helping you improve your technique.

- **Take time to get into the correct starting position** and the rest of the exercise should follow on correctly. Study the photographs and instructions and check yourself against them in case mistakes creep in. Remember if an exercise is done incorrectly you are wasting your efforts and it can even be harmful.

- **Always work at your own level and pace.** Perhaps you will only manage a few repetitions to begin with. This is a far better policy than overworking the muscles and joints, tiring and losing your technique and motivation. Always work to your comfort level. If any of the exercises hurt, *STOP*, immediately; reposition yourself and try again.

- **Keep your movements slow and controlled** when lifting and lowering your legs. Working with precision and control is much more effective than flinging your leg up and down in rapid, jerky movements.

- **Lifting your legs too high is usually a result of an incorrect starting position** and working at speed. The hip joint allows a limited sideways movement. It is within this range that your muscles will work safely and effectively. Taking the leg too high rotates your hip out of position and you end up by working the wrong muscle groups and, worse, your back takes the strain.

Finally, follow my guidelines to ensure pain-free exercising and successful results.

GUIDELINES TO HELP YOU GET THE MOST FROM YOUR EXERCISING

- When you first start, do only *one* exercise for each area—the first illustrated version. When you can comfortably perform all the suggested repetitions and sets (the number of times you perform the repetitions) over a period of weeks, do the second version. Eventually aim to do both. If you're an experienced exerciser, start with the second versions and add in the first when you feel ready.

- **Be balanced.** If you start with the front of your thighs, next, concentrate on the backs. Similarly with the outsides and insides of your thighs. Always include plenty of stretching (turn to pages 33–39 and 55–62 for the specially designed stretching exercises).

- **Repetitions and sets.** When you begin, aim for 10 repetitions (one set) for each exercise and each leg where relevant. When this becomes easier, rest before repeating another set of 10. After a period of several weeks you should be ready to start adding a third set. At this point do all three sets before switching legs and without resting. (For more seasoned exercisers, aim to start off with three sets without switching legs or resting.)

- **Progression.** Aim for the following:
  1 Make the exercise harder by performing the second version, or do both first and second versions
  2 Decrease the rest interval between sets
  3 Add light ankle weights — 0.5–1kg (1–2lb) as long as you have no joint problems
  4 Increase the number of repetitions in the last set

5 Increase the number of days you exercise only as long as you still have 'rest' days

● **Breathing** As a general rule of thumb, breathe **out** on the effort part (that's generally as you perform an exercise) and **in** on the 'release' or return part. Use the whole ribcage — side to side as well as front to back. If you find it difficult to start with, don't worry — just breathe regularly and easily throughout.

STARTER TIPS

- Choose a time when you feel happiest exercising and will have the minimum of interruption.
- Exercise in a warm, light, airy room.
- Wear comfortable, loose clothing and supportive shoes when necessary.
- Although these exercises don't need equipment, a full length mirror is invaluable when checking your positioning and alignment. A mat or towel to lie on offers more comfort and an extra pillow or cushion is a useful aid for some exercises.
- If you feel tired or sore *after* you've exercised, take it easier next time and increase the time you spend stretching and warming down at the end.
- If you do feel pain *during* an exercise, STOP immediately. Readjust your position and continue. If pain persists, stop and seek professional advice.
- Discuss your exercise plans with your doctor if you have had or suffer from any back, neck or joint problems, high blood pressure, heart or chest problems, are pregnant or under medication.
- Finally, start slowly and gradually build up. Don't expect miracles overnight. Be patient and persevere for those great legs!

WARM UP

Never miss out or skimp this part of your exercising whether you decide to exercise at home or in the office or set off for a jog. Always take time to warm up — it only takes about 10 minutes.

Warming up before more demanding activity helps to improve your performance and skill of this activity — it prepares the body by raising body temperature and helps to reduce the risk of injury and soreness. The heart and lungs are also prepared for the main activity to follow.

How to warm up

Include exercises to mobilize and loosen your joints. Move your joints through their normal range of movement but *not* beyond. A warm up also includes stretch exercises. For more stretching ideas, use those illustrated on pages 35–39. Aim to hold each stretch for a count of eight, breathing easily.

Remember to keep all movements free, fluid and flowing. Avoid forced, jerky or too strenuous movements. Remember, it's only the warm up!

Warm down and stretch

Just as you warmed up, so you need to taper off your activity by warming down to induce a feeling of relaxation and well-being. End each session with some rhythmical exercise similar to the warm-up and include plenty of stretches to help reduce the likelihood of post-exercise stiffness and soreness. Repeat the stretching exercises illustrated throughout the book as they have been chosen to correspond directly to the muscle groups you have been exercising. Include the stretch on page 62 liberally throughout your session.

During the warm down, increase the time you hold each stretch by counting up to between 20 and 30, but only hold each position for as long as it feels comfortable. Stretch to the point of mild discomfort but *not* pain. Always breathe easily throughout, never hold your breath.

BEFORE THE OFF — POSTURE POINTERS

Before you start, improve your overall body shape and image by working on your posture. It will also ensure that you start off properly and that you will exercise safely and effectively. Check that:

- your weight is evenly balanced between your feet.
- your insteps are lifted.
- your knees line up over your ankles.
- your hips are level and 'centred'. This means you do a Pelvic Tilt — a simple but effective movement to ensure that your lower back lengthens and the abdominal muscles contract before you do anything else. See page 22 for a fuller explanation of how to do a Pelvic Tilt.
- your shoulders are down and back from your ears and aligned over your ankles.
- your arms hang loosely down by your sides.
- your ribcage lifts up and away from your hips.
- your chest is open by bringing your shoulder blades closer together.
- your head lifts upwards towards the ceiling so that you feel the back of your neck lengthen.
- your chin is at right-angles to the ground.

Always aim for maximum length from the base of your spine to the crown of your head. Feel your entire spine lengthen. Run through these posture pointers and the Pelvic Tilt until you feel confident and happy with the image in your mirror.

Now you're ready to turn the page to start the warm up exercises.

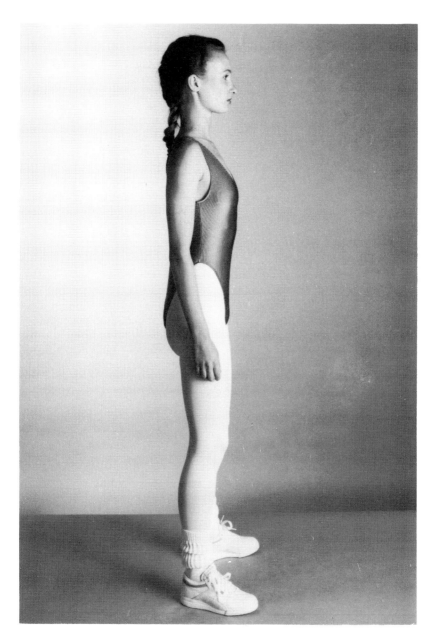

PELVIC TILT

This basic movement ensures that your lower back is protected while you exercise. These instructions are for doing the Pelvic Tilt lying down and it is good to practise in this position but once you have got the hang of it, it can be done in any position.

- Lie on your back on a mat
- Bend your knees and place your feet firmly on the floor so that your legs feel at a comfortable angle
- Pull your shoulders and chin down to lengthen your neck
- Place your right hand on your pubic bone, your left hand under the small of your back
- Breathe out and press your lower back down onto your hand
- Contract your abdominal muscles and feel the upward tilt of your pubic bone against your right hand — try not to squeeze your buttock muscles
- Hold the position, breathing easily
- Release yourself from the position slowly and repeat several times until you feel confident of the movement

Tips: it is only a small movement try not to lift your bottom off the floor

concentrate on contracting or pulling in your abdominal muscles and tilting your pubic bone up

make sure your chin stays level and that your shoulders don't lift

22

ON-THE-SPOT WALKING

- Start by standing well (see Posture Pointers)
- Walk on the spot by transferring your weight from foot to foot, lifting your heels and rolling through to the ball of each foot
- Let your arms swing freely to and fro
- Keep your head lifted, your chin level and your shoulders down
- Gradually increase the pace, letting your arms work freely as if you were marching down the street
- Keep this pace going for one minute, breathing easily

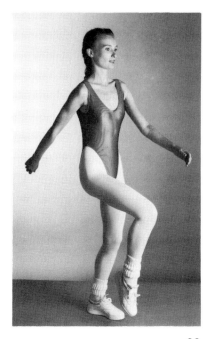

SHOULDERS

- Stand still from marching with your legs about hip-width apart
- Using one count for each movement, lift both your shoulders up, press them gently back and then pull them strongly down
- Repeat fluidly 10 times, breathing easily

Tips: lengthen your neck and back, maintain a Pelvic Tilt,

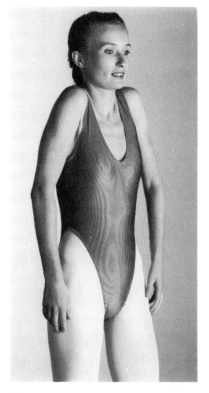
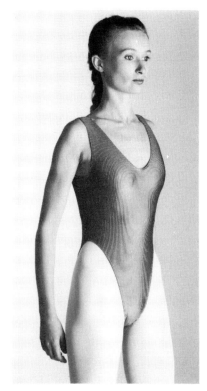

ARM CIRCLES

- Lift your right arm straight out in front of you, brush it gently back past your ear and down to form a complete circle
- Repeat 5 times before doing the same with your left arm
- Repeat a further 5 times using both arms slowly, breathing easily

Tips: maintain a Pelvic Tilt

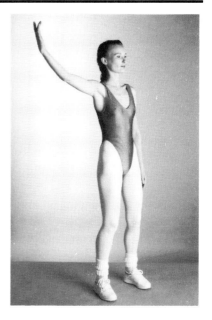

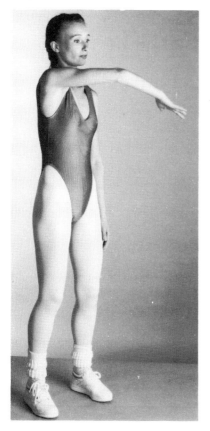

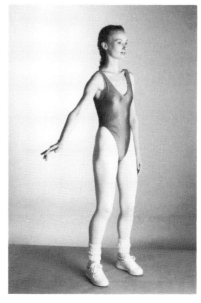

ON-THE-SPOT WALKING

- Repeat this again as described on page 23 for one minute, breathing easily

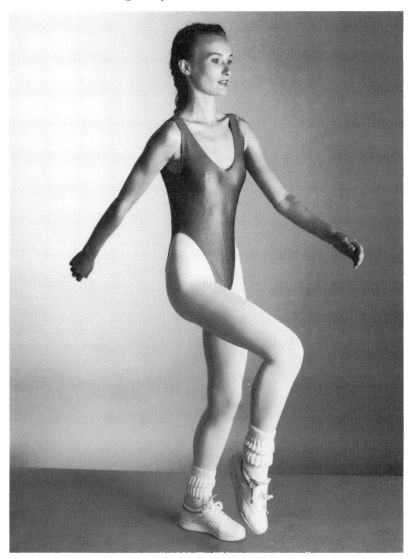

CHEST AND UPPER BACK

- Stand still with your legs about hip-width apart and knees slightly bent
- Take your arms behind your back and interlock your fingers so that they rest just above your bottom
- Squeeze your shoulder blades together so that the gap between your elbows narrows
- Hold for a moment, feeling the stretch across your chest
- Release and repeat twice more, breathing easily

Tips: maintain a Pelvic Tilt keep your shoulders down

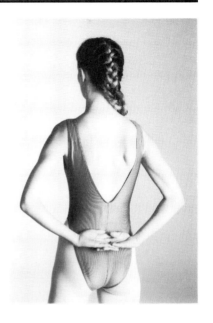

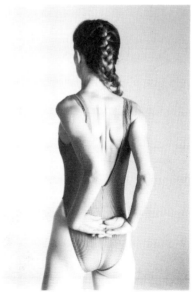

STRETCH AND REACH

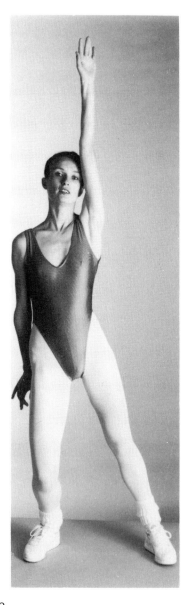

- Stand, maintaining a good posture, with your legs wide apart and your feet slightly turned out
- Bend your knee a little, keeping it lined up over your ankle
- At the same time, stretch your arm up to the ceiling
- Change sides, continuing to bend knees and stretch up, reaching side to side
- Repeat 20 times in a steady and flowing rhythm, breathing easily

Tips: maintain a Pelvic Tilt
pull your shoulders down
keep your head 'centred'

SIDE BENDS

- Stand well with your legs wide apart and, if you prefer, with your knees slightly bent
- Keep a Pelvic Tilt with your hips steady and your shoulders square to the front
- Bend up and out to the left, slowly letting your left hand slide down your thigh for support

- Return slowly to an upright position and repeat the same movement to the right
- Repeat 10 times, 5 each side, breathing easily

Tips: keep your hips still and your abdominal muscles firm check that you don't lean forwards or backwards

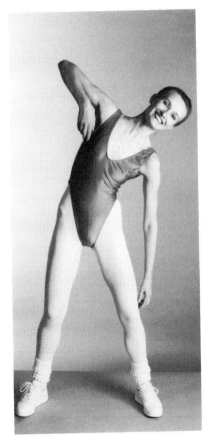
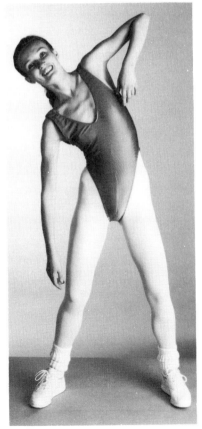

ON-THE-SPOT KNEE LIFTS

- Stand well with your legs almost together
- Start walking on the spot, as shown on page 23, letting your arms swing freely to and fro as if you were marching
- Without changing your posture or balance, lift one knee at a time up to hip level
- Keep this rhythm going for one minute breathing easily

Tips: keep your body upright and balanced

pull your shoulders down and bend at the knee a little as your other leg lifts

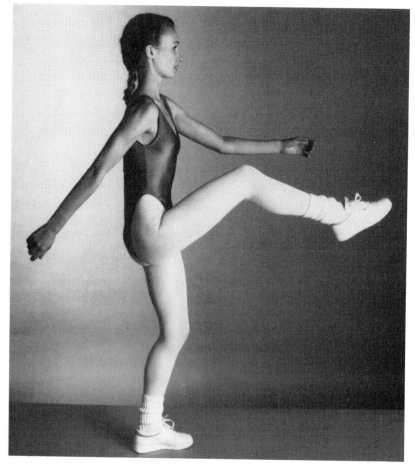

HIP CIRCLES

- Stand well with your legs wide apart and your knees slightly bent over ankles
- Place your hands on your hips
- Move your hips out to one side, carefully round to the back, onto the other side and finally through to the front

- Describe a full circle 10 times to one side and then 10 to the other

Tips: concentrate on your hips, keeping your upper body and legs as still as possible
breathe easily throughout

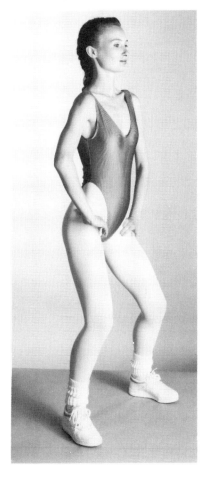
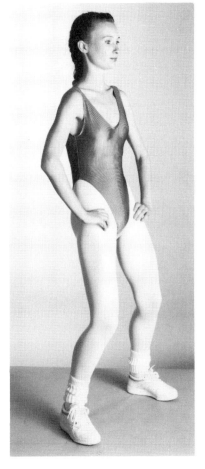

LEGS AND CALVES

- Stand well, holding a firm support
- Open your legs a little wider apart than hip-width, with your feet turned out slightly

- Without changing this posture, bend both your knees a little and line them up over your ankles
- Keep your feet flat as you straighten both your knees

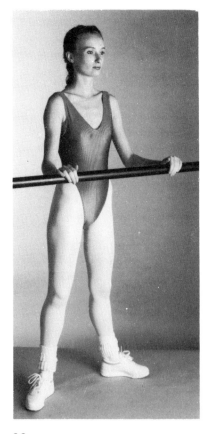 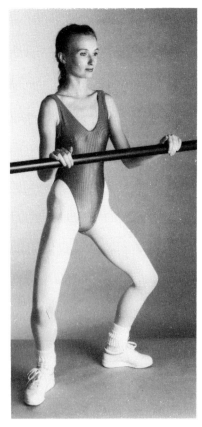

- Now lift both your heels, pausing at the top of the lift before lowering them to the floor

- Continue this rhythm — bend, stretch, lift, lower — until your thighs and calves start to tire
- Breathe easily throughout

Tips: keep the movement fluid and controlled
keep your back long and maintain a Pelvic Tilt

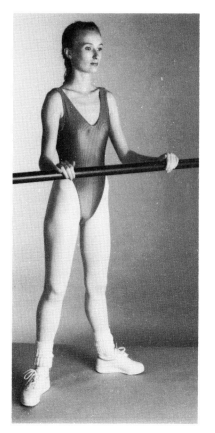
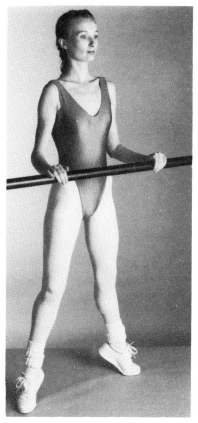

ON-THE-SPOT KNEE LIFTS

- Repeat the exercise as described on page 26 for one minute, breathing easily

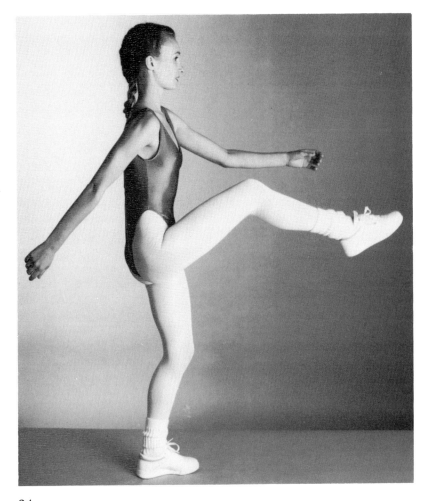

CALF STRETCH 1

- Stand well, holding a firm support with your legs close together
- Without changing posture, slide your right foot straight back behind you in line with your hip until you feel a stretch in your calf
- Make sure your foot is firmly in place and press your heel down
- Bend your left knee slightly over your ankle
- Hold the position for a slow count of 8, breathing easily

- Feel the stretch in the calf of your right leg
- Release the stretch slowly and then repeat with your left leg

Tips: keep a Pelvic Tilt and your hips square to the front
pull your shoulders down
keep both your feet flat on the floor and facing straight ahead

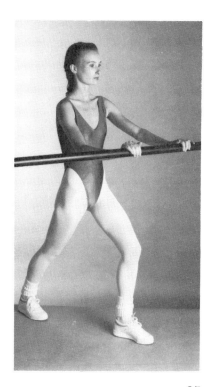

CALF STRETCH 2

- Stand as before, with your right leg behind you, in line with your hip and press your heel down into the floor
- Bend your left knee slightly over your ankle
- Maintaining this position, bend your right knee slightly and continue pressing your heel down into the floor
- Hold for a slow count of 8, breathing easily
- Feel the stretch lower down in the calf of your right leg
- Release yourself slowly from this position and then repeat for your left

Tips: As for calf stretch 1

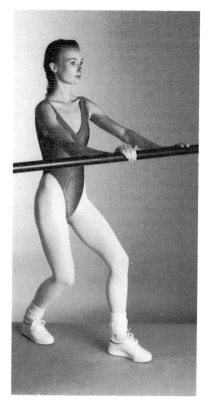

FRONT THIGH STRETCH

- Stand well, holding a firm support
- Without changing your posture, bring your right foot back up towards your bottom
- Use your right hand to gently pull your feet in closer to your bottom
- Hold this position for a slow count of 8, breathing easily

- Feel the stretch at the front of your thigh
- Release yourself from this position slowly, and repeat with your left leg

Tips: keep a Pelvic Tilt and keep your back long
stop if you feel pain in or around the knee joint

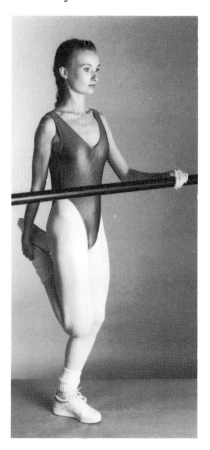

INSIDE THIGH STRETCH

- Sit so that your back and neck are long and, if necessary, sit up against a wall for support
- Bring the soles of your feet together
- Rest your hands on your ankles (without pulling on them)
- Vary the position of your feet and knees until you feel a stretch along the insides of your thighs and your groin
- Hold for a slow count of 8, breathing easily
- Release yourself from this position slowly

Tips: keep your back long and pull your shoulders down
if you feel pain in or around your knees, *stop*

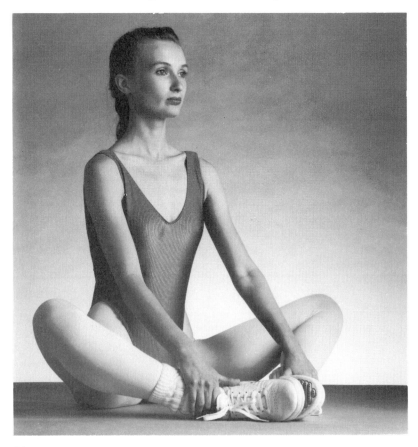

BACK OF THIGH STRETCH

- Lie on your back on a mat (not shown)
- Bend your knees and then place your feet flat on the floor so your knees are at a comfortable angle
- Hold the back of your left thigh and pull it down towards your chest
- Slowly stretch your leg towards the ceiling
- Hold this position for slow count of 8, breathing easily
- Feel a stretch at back of your thigh

- Release yourself slowly from this position and then repeat the exercise for your right leg

Tips: keep your lower back pressing into the floor
check that your opposite knee doesn't move out to one side
pull your shoulders down and keep your chin in

Now you are warmed up and ready to move on to the main exercises

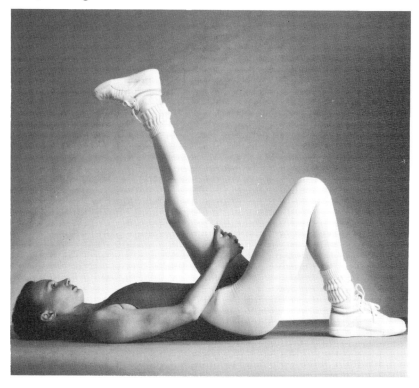

THE MAIN EXERCISES

When you are first starting out, begin with the first exercise for each part of the legs. Progress to the next exercise for each part of the legs and then when you are ready, include both in your exercise session.

Tips: keep your chin in and down
keep your lower back on your hands by holding your abdominal muscles firm
pull your shoulders down from your ears
aim to fully straighten your leg *without* it dropping forwards

FRONT OF THIGH TIGHTENERS

- Lie flat on your back on a mat (not shown)
- Place both your hands under your bottom
- Bring your thighs, one at a time, into your chest
- Slowly straighten your right leg up towards the ceiling
- Pause, breathing easily, at the topmost position
- Feel the front of your thigh tighten and the back of your leg stretch
- Return to your starting position
- Repeat for your left leg until you have worked up to 10 repetitions on each leg (gradually build up to second and third sets)

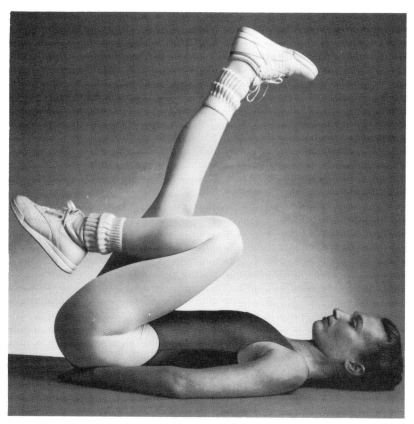

41

FRONT THIGH LIFTS

- Sit on a mat (not shown) with your back long and, if necessary, up against a firm support
- Bend your left leg in towards your chest
- Rest your hand by your sides or grasp below your bent knee to help you maintain your posture
- Stretch your right leg straight out in front of you
- Pull your toes back up towards the ceiling without 'locking' your knee

- Slowly lift your right leg off the floor and then lower it again
- Feel the front of your thigh tighten as you lift
- Repeat up to 10 times for each leg, working towards second and third sets

Tips: keep your hips still and your lower back supported
use a pillow in the small of your back for comfort, if necessary
relax your upper body

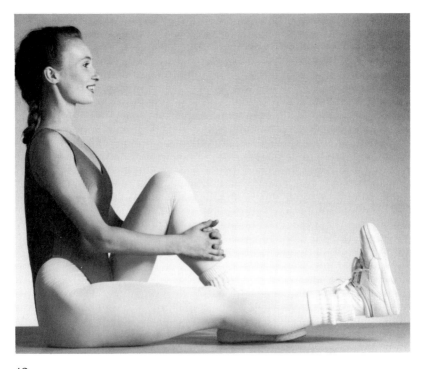

BACK OF THIGH CURLS

- Lie on your front on a mat (not shown) in a straight line
- Rest your forehead on your hands
- Press your hips down onto the mat and tighten your bottom muscles throughout the exercise
- Slowly bring your right foot up towards your bottom, keeping your thigh on the floor
- Pause, breathing easily before slowly lowering your leg back towards the floor
- Feel the back of your thigh tighten as your foot draws closer to your bottom
- Repeat with your left leg until you have worked up to 10 repetitions for each leg (gradually build up to second and third sets)

Tips: keep your movements slow and controlled

keep your upper body still and relaxed

stop if you feel knee pain and try lifting your leg straight, keeping hips pressed into the floor

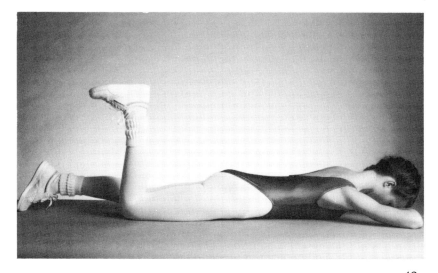

KNEELING/BACK OF THIGH LIFTS

- Kneel on all fours on a mat (not shown)
- Shift your weight slightly forward by lowering yourself onto your elbows
- Do a Pelvic Tilt and contract your abdominal muscles
- Bring your right foot up towards your buttock
- Tighten your buttocks and slowly lift your knee to just below the level of your hips
- Pause, breathing easily before slowly lowering your leg to the height of your left calf
- Feel the back of your thighs and buttocks tighten as your knee lifts

- Repeat up to 10 times for each leg, working gradually towards being able to complete second and third sets

Tips: don't arch your lower back or turn your hips out to gain more height

keep your hips still and square to the floor

keep your head aligned with your back

keep your body-weight centred — don't collapse on your supporting side

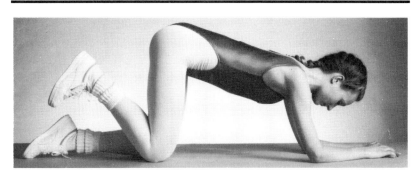

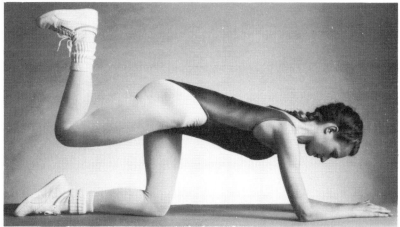

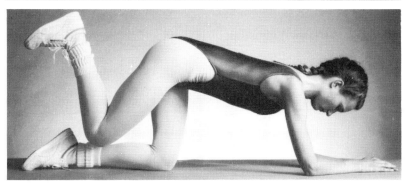

OUTER THIGH LIFTS LYING ON YOUR SIDE

- Lie on your left side in a straight line on a mat (not shown)
- Rest your head on your hand and rest your other hand palm down in front of you for more support
- Bend your left leg
- Look down the front of your body and check that you form one continuous line
- Keep your hips square and your abdominal muscles firm
- Slowly lift your right leg, pulling your foot back towards your face without 'locking' your knee
- Pause, breathing easily, at the topmost position before slowly lowering your leg, stopping a little way above the floor
- Feel your leg tighten into your hip as it lifts
- Repeat up to 10 times for each leg (gradually build up to second and third sets)

Tips: keep your weight slightly forwards and don't roll back as your leg lifts

keep your knee, hip and foot facing straight ahead

if your neck tires, rest your head on your arm

if you prefer, only bring your lifting leg halfway up

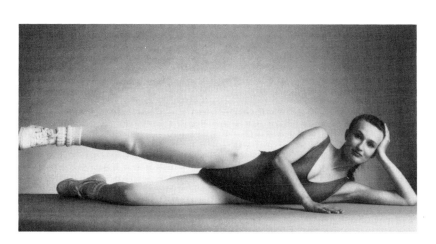

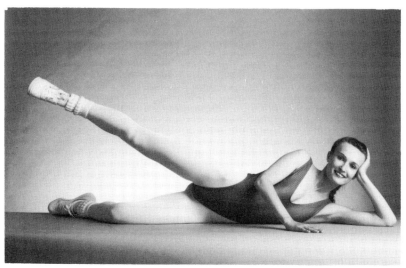

BENT THIGH LIFTS

- Start in the same position as for Outer thigh lifts lying on your side, but bend your knees to form right angles to your body
- Keep your knees and feet in line
- Keep your abdominal muscles firm throughout
- Slowly lift your right leg to line up with your hip
- Pause, breathing easily, at the topmost position before slowly lowering your leg again, stopping before it touches your left leg
- Feel your outside thigh muscles working when you are lifting your leg
- Repeat the exercise up to 10 times for each leg, working towards being able to add second and third sets

Tips: don't let your top hip roll back as you lift your leg

keep your whole leg moving as one unit — don't let your lower leg waggle

if this position doesn't suit your back, align your legs at a 45 degree angle so that your thighs slope away from your hips

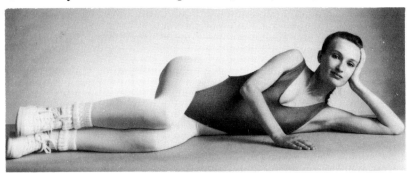

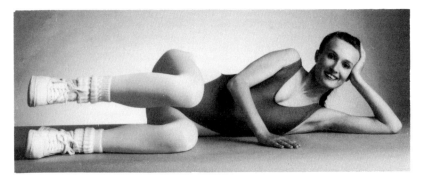

INSIDE THIGH SQUEEZES

- Lie flat on your back on a mat (not shown)
- Bend your knees, keep your feet flat on the floor and hip-width apart in a comfortable, firm position
- Place a cushion or ball between your inner thighs
- Inch your feet closer together
- Press your lower back into the floor — holding your abdominal muscles firm
- Slowly squeeze your inner thighs together and then relax
- Feel the insides of your thighs tighten as you squeeze them together
- Repeat 10 times, gradually building up to second and third sets
- Breathe easily throughout

Tips: concentrate on the inner thigh action, making sure your bottom doesn't do the work
squeeze the whole length of the inside of your thighs
keep your shoulders relaxed
make sure your lower back doesn't arch when you're working

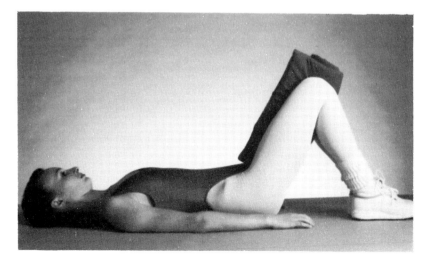

INSIDE THIGH LIFTS

- Lie on your side on a mat (not shown)
- Rest your head on your hand and rest your other hand palm down in front of you for support
- Bring your right leg forwards and rest it on the floor, or if you prefer, keep that knee up
- Straighten your left leg along the floor — pulling your foot back towards your face, keeping your knee and foot facing square to front
- Lift your left leg in one straight line and then repeat little lifts, breathing easily
- Feel the inside of your left thigh tighten as it lifts
- Repeat up to 10 times for each leg, gradually working towards second and third sets

Tips: check that your body forms one continuous line

keep your abdominal muscles firm

if you prefer, you can place several cushions under your top knee to keep it lined up with your top hip

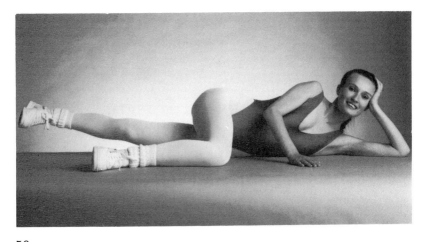

LOWER LEG WARM UP 1

- Stand or sit so that your back and neck are long and relaxed (if you're standing, you may need to hold onto a firm support)
- Keeping your weight balanced and 'centred' lift your left leg slightly out in front of you

- Slowly describe a clockwise circle with your foot 10 times
- Repeat with your other leg
- Reverse the direction as you repeat once more for each foot

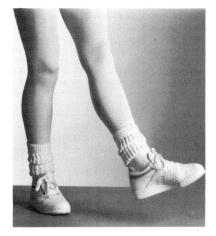 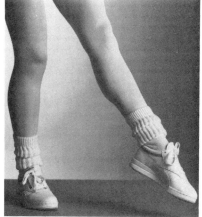

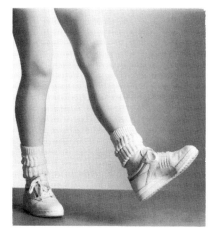 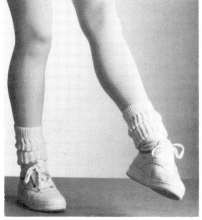

LOWER LEG WARM UP 2

- Start in the same position as for Lower leg warm up 1
- Pull your foot strongly up towards your face and then push it back down again
- Repeat 10 times before repeating with your right leg

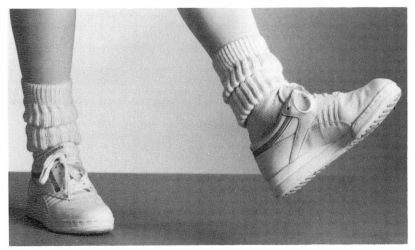

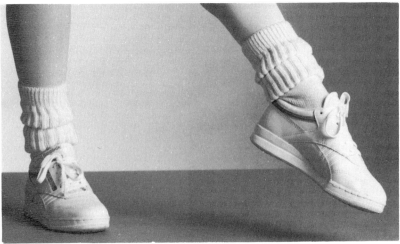

HEEL LIFTS

- Stand, holding a firm support
- Place a block of wood or thick book on the floor — ensuring that it won't slip
- Balance the balls of your feet on the wood or book and ensure that your heels are level with it
- Lift your heels as high as you can and then lower them again without touching the floor with them or bending your knees, breathing easily
- Feel your calf muscles tighten as you lift your heels
- Repeat 10 times and gradually build up to second and third sets

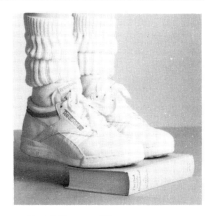

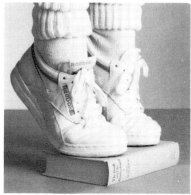

Tips: keep your toes pointing straight ahead and make sure that your ankles don't roll in or out

although you shouldn't bend your knees, make sure they're not 'locked'

keep your body upright, your abdominal and buttock muscles firm and shoulders down and relaxed

to improve your balance, practise without support

TOE TAPS

- Sit or stand so that your back and neck are long and relaxed
- Keep your body-weight balanced and 'centred' throughout
- Lift the toes of your left foot as high as you can without lifting your heel as well
- Tap the front rhythmically on the floor until the front of your lower leg begins to tire
- Repeat with your right leg
- Breathe easily throughout the exercise

Tips always do the Lower leg warm ups before toe taps and end by pointing and flexing

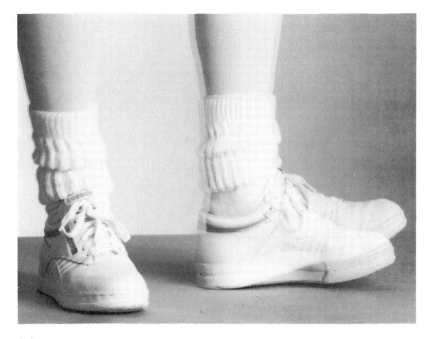

FRONT OF THIGH STRETCH

- Stand well, holding a firm support
- Without changing your posture bring your right foot back up to your bottom
- Keep your knee facing down and in line with your hips
- Hold onto your ankle to increase the stretch
- Feel the stretch along the front of your thigh
- Hold the position, breathing easily, and count slowly between 20 and 30
- Release yourself from the position slowly and repeat with your left leg

Tips keep your bottom 'tucked' under and your chest lifted
stop if you feel pain in or around your knee joint

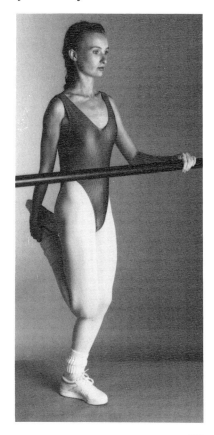

CALF STRETCH 1

- Stand well holding a firm support
- Move your right leg straight out behind your hip without changing your posture.
- Press your heel into the floor
- Bend your front knee over your ankle
- Aim to keep your body-weight 'centred'
- Hold the position, breathing easily, and slowly count between 20 and 30
- Feel the stretch along the calf of your back leg

- Release yourself slowly from this position and repeat for your left leg

Tips: keep your hips level and facing square to the front
pull your shoulders down and tuck your bottom under
keep both your feet flat on the floor and face straight ahead

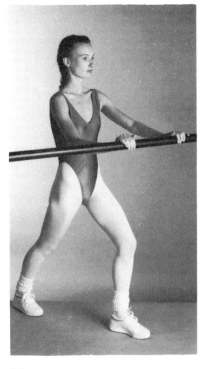

CALF STRETCH 2

- Take up the same position described for Calf stretch 1
- Bend your right knee slightly, pressing your heel down into the floor
- Hold the position, breathing easily and slowly count between 20 and 30
- Feel the stretch lower down in your calf
- Release yourself slowly from the position and repeat for your left leg

Tips: keep your hips level and facing square to the front
pull your shoulders down and tuck your bottom under
keep both your feet flat and facing straight ahead

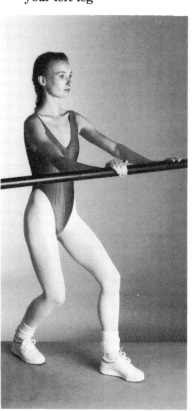

OUTSIDE THIGH STRETCH AND SPINAL TWIST

- Sit upright with both legs straight out in front of you
- Cross your right foot to the outside of your left leg
- Lengthen your back and slowly turn your upper body round to the right
- Place your right hand behind you on the floor for support
- Use your left arm to gently pull your right thigh closer to your chest
- Lengthen your back again as you turn to the right as far as is comfortable
- Feel the stretch along the outside of your right thigh and hip

- Hold the position, breathing easily, and slowly count between 20 and 30
- Release yourself from this position slowly and repeat for your left side, remembering to reverse your leg and arm positions

Tips: turn your head, neck and upper body slowly as one unit
aim to twist your shoulders away from the front to the side
keep your hips and knees facing square to the front
pull your shoulders down and keep your back long

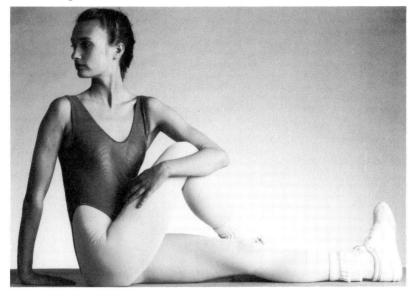

GROIN STRETCH

- Lie on your back on a mat (not shown)
- Hold the back of your right thigh and pull it in towards your chest
- Slowly stretch your left leg along the floor, pulling your foot back up towards you, keeping your leg on the floor
- Keep your lower back and the back of your knee on the floor
- Feel the stretch at the top of your left leg and around the bottom of your right leg
- Hold the position, breathing easily, and count slowly between 20 and 30
- Release yourself from the position slowly and repeat to stretch your right leg

Tips: keep your chin and shoulders down

bring the leg you are clasping closer to your chest *only* if your lower back and extended leg remain flat on the floor

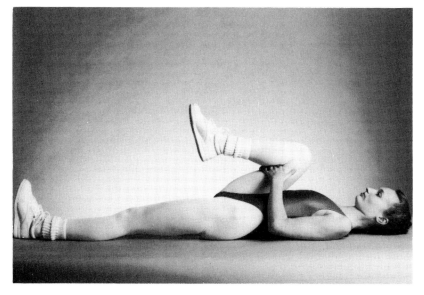

BACK-OF-THIGH STRETCH

- Lie on your back on a mat (not shown)
- Bend your right knee and put your foot flat on the floor so your knee is at a comfortable angle
- Hold the back of your left thigh and pull it in towards your chest
- Slowly stretch your leg towards the ceiling
- Feel a stretch at the back of your thigh
- Hold the position, breathing easily, and slowly count between 20 and 30
- Release yourself from the position slowly and repeat for your right leg

Tips keep your chin down to maintain length in your neck
pull your shoulders down
keep your lower back pressing down into the floor
check that your bent knee doesn't fall to one side

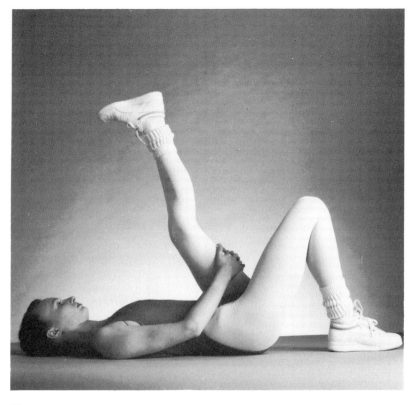

INSIDE THIGH STRETCH

- Lie on your back on a mat (not shown)
- Bend your knees, keeping your feet flat on the floor and rest them at a comfortable angle
- Pull your shoulders down from your ears and rest your arms by your sides
- Slowly lower both your knees out to each side, down to the floor
- Keep the soles of your feet touching and your lower back pressing into the floor
- Hold this position, breathing easily, and slowly count between 20 and 30
- Release yourself from the position by bringing both your knees back up together

Tips: adjust the position of your legs so that they are either more or less bent so that you feel a stretch along your inner thighs and up into your groin

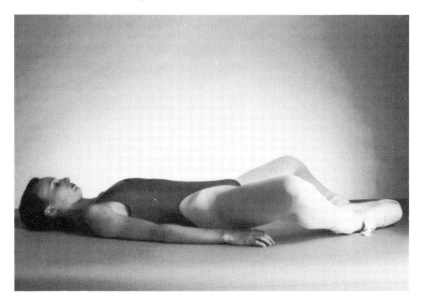

THIGH HUGS

- Lie on your back on a mat (not shown)
- Bring each leg, one at a time, towards your chest
- Hold the backs of your thighs, breathing easily
- Gently hug your thighs closer in to your chest
- Release them a little and repeat as many times as feels comfortable
- To stand up, slowly roll over to one side and sit up using your hands

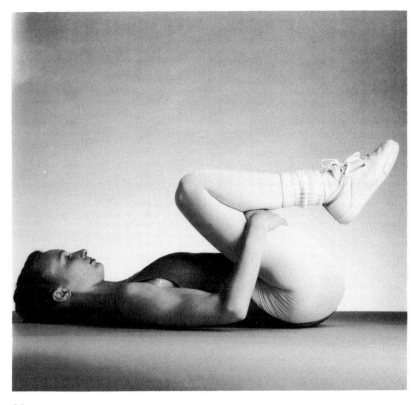

If you would like to take classes with Julia Swift, she can be contacted at the following addresses:

The Old Slipper Baths,
North Road,
Brighton
East Sussex BN1 1YA

Tel: 0273 690016

The Mercury Lower Studio
4 Ladbroke Road,
London W11

Tel: 01-289 0494 (office hours only)